STRETCHING

EXERCISES FOR SENIORS

Over 60

Simple and Effective Stretching Strategies for Older Adults to Improve Posture, Mobility and Decrease Back pain.

....

Dr. Bryant D Baldwin

Table Of Contents

Scan the code to join our 30 day workout challenge also access Stretching Video training for seniors

*How To Scan

1. Navigate to your phone Camera or QR Code Scanner app
2. Centre the code in the space given

3. With your mobile data on you'll be directed to the bonus site.

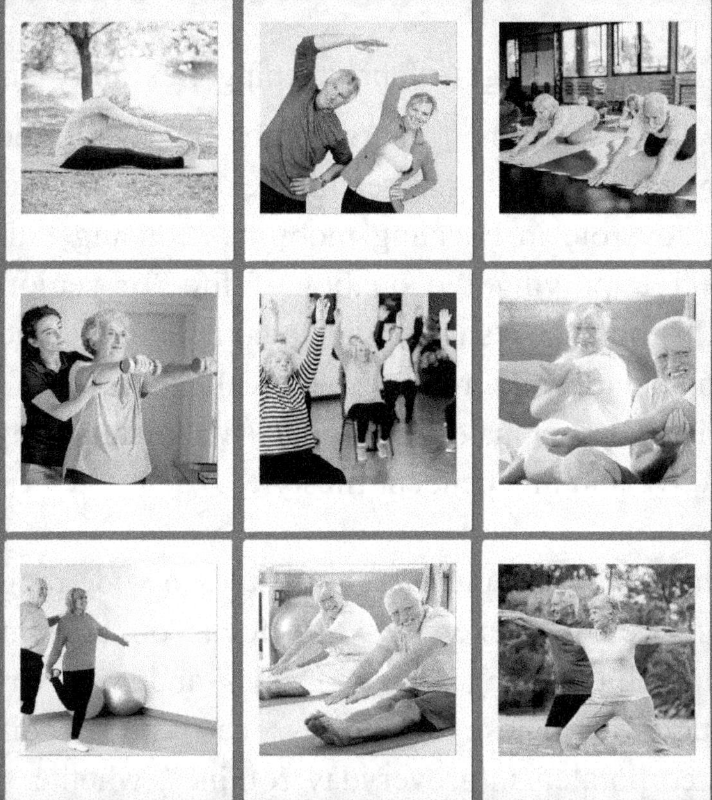

Safe and Easy exercises to make you feel better

INTRODUCTION

As we get older, keeping flexibility and balance becomes increasingly vital for our overall well-being. Stretching exercises can play a key role in boosting mobility, reducing falls, and improving the quality of life for seniors. This book seeks to provide a complete reference to balance exercises specifically created for older individuals, helping them maintain an active and independent lifestyle.

In the next chapters, we will study a wide range of stretching exercises that focus on boosting flexibility, strengthening muscles, and improving stability. These exercises can be readily incorporated into everyday routines, whether at home or in a training set and are adapted to match the special requirements and skills of seniors.

By engaging in regular stretching activities, seniors can experience several benefits, such as greater joint range of motion, reduced muscle stiffness, improved posture, and enhanced blood circulation. Moreover, these activities contribute to a stronger sense of confidence and self-assurance, minimizing the risk of falls and generating a greater sense of general well-being.

It's crucial to approach stretching exercises for seniors with care and deliberation, taking into account individual physical abilities, medical problems, and any potential limits. Therefore, this book will include precise directions, variations, and safety tips to ensure a safe and successful stretching program for seniors of all fitness levels.

Whether you are a senior trying to maintain or enhance your balance, a caregiver supporting an older loved one, or a fitness expert working with older persons, this book will serve as a great resource for introducing balancing exercises into daily life.

Benefits of Stretching for Seniors

Stretching exercises offer a range of benefits for seniors, helping to improve their entire physical and mental well-being. Here are some significant advantages of including stretching into the everyday routine of older adults:

1. Improved Flexibility: As we age, our muscles and joints tend to become less flexible, resulting in a reduced range of motion and greater stiffness. Regular stretching can counteract this by increasing flexibility and joint mobility, allowing elderly to move with greater ease and comfort.

2. Enhanced Balance and Stability: Balance exercises are vital for reducing falls, a significant worry among seniors. Stretching practices that target the muscles involved in maintaining balance, such as the legs and core, can assist improve stability and lower

the chance of falls, thus fostering greater independence and confidence.

3. Reduced Muscle Tension and Pain: Aging bodies commonly feel muscle tension and discomfort. Stretching exercises can ease muscle tension, enhance blood circulation, and reduce stiffness, providing relief from aches and pains frequently linked with aging.

4. Improved Posture: Poor posture can contribute to several health ailments, including back discomfort and decreased mobility. Stretching helps lengthen tight muscles and strengthen weak ones, improving posture and alignment, and minimizing the risk of postural issues.

5. Increased Energy and Vitality: Engaging in regular stretching practices improves blood flow, bringing oxygen and nutrients to the muscles and organs. This improved circulation can boost energy levels, improve mood, and create a general sense of vigor and well-being.

6. Stress Relief and Relaxation: Stretching exercises can have a relaxing effect on the mind and body. By focusing on slow, controlled movements and deep breathing, seniors can enjoy a sense of relaxation and stress reduction, boosting their overall mental health.

Safety Considerations for Senior Stretching

While stretching is generally safe and useful for seniors, it is vital to prioritize safety and take basic precautions to prevent injury. Here are some crucial safety precautions to bear in mind when partaking in stretching exercises:

1. Consult with a Healthcare Professional: Before starting any new fitness regimen, seniors need to consult with their healthcare professional. They can provide significant insights and suggestions depending on

specific health problems, medications, and physical restrictions.

2. Warm-Up Before Stretching: It is vital to warm up the body before stretching to enhance blood flow to the muscles and prepare them for exercise. Gentle cardiovascular movements like walking or stationary cycling for a few minutes can help warm up the body.

3. Start Slow and Progress progressively: Seniors should begin with mild stretches and progressively increase the intensity and duration over time. Avoid jumping or jerking motions, as they might strain muscles and joints. Slow and controlled motions are crucial to safe and successful stretching.

4. Listen to Your Body: Seniors should pay attention to their bodies and avoid pushing beyond their comfort zones. Mild discomfort during stretching is normal, but sharp or

intense pain should be a cue to pause and reassess the activity.

5. Use Proper Technique: Proper form and technique are vital to minimize injury and optimize the benefits of stretching. Seniors should follow directions attentively, maintain good alignment, and avoid excessive strain on joints and muscles.

6. Modify Exercises as Needed: Seniors with certain physical limitations or conditions may need to modify certain stretches. It is crucial to find variants or alternatives that are safe and fit for individual requirements and abilities.

7. Stay Hydrated: Hydration is vital for overall health, even during stretching activities. Seniors should drink lots of water before, during, and after their stretching practices to prevent dehydration and promote optimal muscular function.

Understanding Aging and Flexibility

Our bodies naturally endure changes that can influence flexibility As we age. Muscles may grow tighter, joints may lose some range of motion, and connective tissues may become less elastic. However, it's crucial to note that keeping flexibility with regular stretching exercises can help counteract these consequences, boosting mobility, reducing stiffness, and raising the general quality of life.

How Aging Affects Flexibility

Aging can greatly decrease flexibility due to several physiological changes that occur in the body. Here are several important ways in which aging decreases flexibility:

1. Reduced Muscle Elasticity: With age, muscles tend to lose their elasticity, making them less malleable and more prone to stiffness. This decrease in elasticity can inhibit joint movement and reduce overall flexibility.

2. Increased Connective Tissue Stiffness: The connective tissues in our bodies, such as tendons and ligaments, become less flexible and more rigid over time. This diminished flexibility in the connective tissues might further lead to restrictions in joint mobility and range of motion.

3. Joint Degeneration: As we age, the cartilage that cushions your joints may wear down, leading to joint degeneration and an increased risk of disorders such as osteoarthritis. This

can cause discomfort, irritation, and stiffness, further limiting flexibility.

4. Loss of Muscle Mass: Age-related muscle loss, known as sarcopenia, can result in weakening muscles and diminished strength. Weaker muscles can decrease flexibility and make it tougher to perform specific activities with ease.

5. Postural Changes: Aging can lead to changes in posture, such as rounding of the spine or forward head posture. These postural abnormalities might impact muscle length and flexibility, resulting in a restricted range of motion.

Common Flexibility Issues in Seniors

Seniors often suffer special flexibility concerns due to the natural aging process and lifestyle variables. Here are some frequent flexibility concerns reported by seniors:

1. Limited Joint Range of Motion: Aging can lead to diminished joint mobility and flexibility, making it tougher to accomplish routine activities that require bending, reaching, or twisting.

2. Stiffness in the Lower Back: Many seniors have stiffness and tightness in the lower back, which can be linked to age-related changes, sedentary lifestyles, or previous injuries. This can compromise movement and overall flexibility.

3. Tightness in the Hips: Tight hip muscles are a typical condition among seniors. This tightness can hinder movement, compromise balance, and raise the risk of falls.

4. Decreased Flexibility in the Shoulders: Aging can cause a loss of flexibility in the shoulders, making it challenging to make overhead movements, reach behind the back,

or engage in activities that demand a wide range of shoulder motion.

5. Tight Leg Muscles: Seniors commonly experience tightness in the muscles of the legs, including the hamstrings, quadriceps, and calves. This tightness can limit mobility, impair gait patterns, and raise the risk of muscular strains or accidents.

6. Limited Spinal Mobility: Age-related changes, such as degenerative disc disease or spinal arthritis, can contribute to decreased spinal flexibility. This can impair posture, overall movement, and daily activities.

Addressing these common flexibility difficulties with regular stretching exercises can help seniors increase their range of motion, reduce stiffness, and boost their overall flexibility, leading to improved functional capacity and a higher quality of life.

Chapter 1

Getting Started: Preparing for Stretching

Before entering into a stretching regimen, it's necessary to prepare your body for the workouts ahead. Start by warming up with modest aerobic activities like walking or cycling to enhance blood flow and loosen muscles. Gather any essential equipment, choose a comfortable area, and mentally focus on the impending stretching practice for the best results.

Warm-up Exercises

A full warm-up is crucial before engaging in stretching activities, especially for seniors. It helps boost blood flow to the muscles, raise body temperature, and prepare the body for physical exertion. Here are four great warm-up routines for seniors:

1. Marching in Place

Stand tall with feet hip-width apart. Lift your right leg as high as comfortable while swinging your left arm forward, then repeat with the left knee and right arm. Continue alternating legs for 1-2 minutes, gradually increasing the tempo.

2. Shoulder Rolls

Stand or sit erect with arms relaxed by your sides. Slowly roll your shoulders forward in a circular motion, making huge circles. Repeat for 10-15 rotations, then reverse the direction and roll them backward.

3. Ankle Circles

Sit comfortably in a chair and lift one foot off the ground. Rotate your foot clockwise in a circular manner, then switch to counterclockwise. Perform 5-10 circles in each direction, then switch to the other foot.

4. Arm Swings

Stand with feet shoulder-width apart. Extend your arms straight out to the sides, parallel to the floor. Swing your arms forth and backward in a controlled manner, gradually increasing the range of motion. Perform 10-15 swings in each direction.

Equipment & Tools for Stretching

While stretching exercises can be done without any equipment, various tools and props can enhance the efficiency and comfort of the stretches. Here are some popular equipment and instruments for stretching:

1. Exercise Mat: An exercise mat provides a nice and cushioned surface for floor-based stretching exercises. It helps protect joints and gives stability during stretching activities.

2. Resistance Bands: Resistance bands are useful instruments that may add resistance to stretches, helping to develop strength and flexibility. They come in varying levels of resistance, allowing seniors to adapt their workouts according to their skills.

3. Foam Roller: A foam roller is a cylindrical foam tool used for self-massage and myofascial relief. It can help reduce muscle tension, promote flexibility, and improve mobility. Seniors can use a foam roller to target specific muscle regions and boost their stretching practices.

4. Yoga Blocks: Yoga blocks are supportive tools used to alter and deepen practices. They give support and help elderly maintain good

alignment during stretches, especially if they have limited flexibility or balance.

5. Stability Ball: A stability ball can be used for stretching activities that demand balance and core engagement. It adds an element of instability, testing the muscles and developing flexibility and strength.

6. Towel or Strap: A towel or strap can be used to assist with stretching exercises, especially for people with poor flexibility. It can be used to reach for the feet, hold stretches, or assist in stretching the upper body.

While equipment and tools might enhance your stretching experience, they are not required. Seniors can still get excellent stretches utilizing just their bodies and a safe, comfortable setting. It's crucial to choose equipment that meets individual demands, preferences, and physical ability.

Chapter 2

Stretching Techniques for Seniors

Stretching is a helpful technique for seniors to preserve flexibility and increase mobility. Here are some helpful stretching practices for elderly adults:

Static Stretching

Static stretching is a popular and regularly used stretching technique that involves keeping a stretch in a stationary position for a specific length, often between 15 and 30 seconds. During static stretching, the muscle is stretched to a point of mild tension and held without any bouncing or jerking movements. This approach tries to enhance flexibility by gradually elongating the muscles and increasing their range of motion. Static stretching is commonly performed after a warm-up or as part of a cool-down practice. It helps to relax the muscles, alleviate muscle stiffness, and enhance general flexibility. Examples of static stretches are hamstring stretches, shoulder stretches, and calf stretches.

Dynamic Stretching

Dynamic stretching entails performing controlled, repetitive movements that take a joint or muscle through its full range of motion. Unlike static stretching, dynamic stretching comprises active movements that replicate the motions required during physical activities or workouts. This technique is particularly effective for warming up the body before engaging in more strenuous exercises. Dynamic stretches help to enhance blood flow, elevate heart rate, and prepare the muscles and joints for exercise. They also promote flexibility, enhance coordination, and improve athletic performance. Examples of dynamic stretches for seniors may include arm swings, leg swings, and trunk rotations.

Proprioceptive Neuromuscular Facilitation (PNF) Stretching

Proprioceptive Neuromuscular Facilitation (PNF) stretching is an advanced stretching technique that utilizes a combination of tightening and relaxing muscles to enhance flexibility. PNF stretching often requires a partner or the use of a strap or towel for support.

The technique normally involves three phases: stretching the target muscle, an isometric contraction of the muscle against resistance, and then a passive stretch with the support of a partner. PNF stretching employs the body's neuromuscular responses to achieve a broader range of motion and improve muscle flexibility.
It is often utilized in rehabilitative and sports performance settings to enhance flexibility and improve muscular strength and control.

Active Isolated Stretching (AIS)

Active Isolated Stretching (AIS) is a stretching technique that involves the active engagement of the muscles being stretched. In AIS, each stretch is performed for a short length, usually 1-2 seconds, and then released. After a brief pause, the stretch is done numerous times.

The purpose of AIS is to promote flexibility and range of motion by using the opposing muscles to actively bring the target muscle into a stretch. This approach helps to lengthen muscles, promote joint mobility, and improve muscular coordination. AIS is widely used by athletes and anyone trying to enhance overall flexibility and prevent injuries.

When implementing any stretching technique, it is crucial to emphasize safety and listen to your body. Start with mild stretches and progressively build intensity and duration over time.

It is also essential to check with a healthcare practitioner or a trained fitness instructor, especially if you have any specific health problems or physical restrictions. Remember to warm up before stretching and to maintain appropriate form and technique throughout the stretching exercises.

Stretching Exercises for the Upper Body

Maintaining flexibility in the upper body is critical for seniors to improve posture, ease tension, and promote range of motion. Effective upper body stretches include shoulder rolls, arm crossovers, triceps stretches, and neck stretches. Perform these exercises daily to increase upper body flexibility and overall well-being.

Neck Stretches

1. Neck Tilt

Sit or stand erect, then gradually tilt your head to one side, bringing your ear nearer your shoulder. Hold the stretch for 15-30 seconds, then repeat on the opposite side.

2. Neck Rotation

Slowly turn your head to one side, attempting to put your chin over your shoulder. Hold for 15-30 seconds and repeat on the opposite side.

3. Neck Flexion

Lower your chin toward your chest, experiencing a stretch down the back of your neck. Hold for 15-30 seconds, then slowly return to a neutral posture.

4. Neck Extension

Gently tilt your head backward, looking up towards the ceiling. Feel the stretch in the front of your neck and hold for 15-30 seconds. Return to a neutral position.

5. Neck Retraction

Sit or stand with proper posture. Slowly drag your chin inside, forming a double chin. Hold for a few seconds, then release. Repeat for multiple repetitions.

Shoulder and Arm Stretches

1. **Cross-Body Arm Stretch**

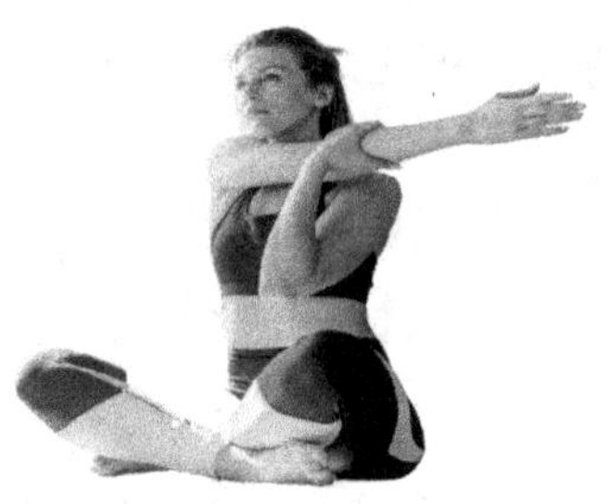

Extend one arm across your chest and use the opposing hand to gently draw it closer to your body, experiencing a stretch in the shoulder and upper back. Hold for 15-30 seconds and repeat on the opposite side.

2. **Triceps Stretch**

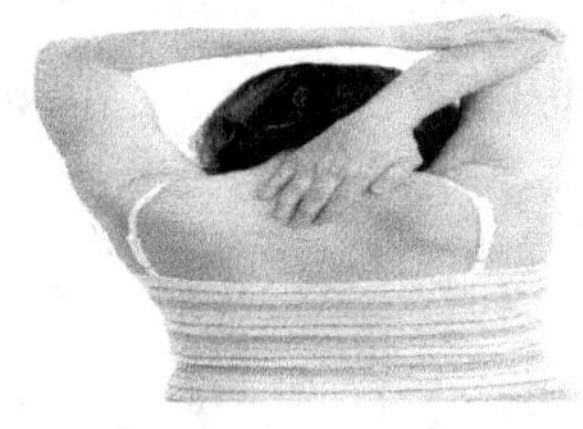

Extend one arm overhead and bend your elbow, stretching your hand towards the opposite shoulder blade. Use your other hand to gently press the elbow further if needed. Hold for 15-30 seconds and repeat on the opposite side.

3. Bicep Stretch

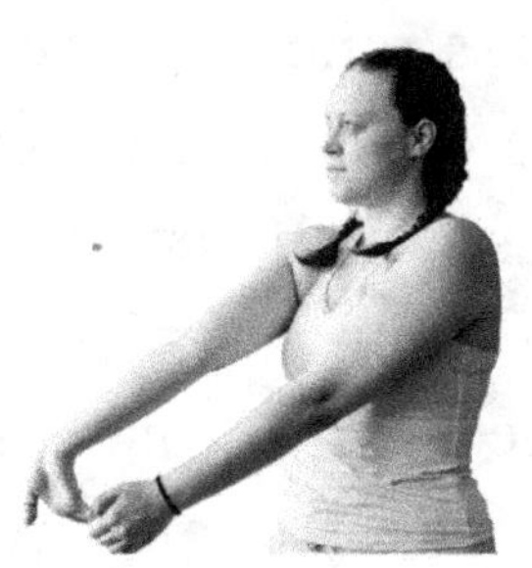

Stand or sit with proper posture.

Extend one arm straight in front of you, palm facing upward. Use the opposite hand to slowly pull the fingers back, experiencing a stretch in the bicep. Hold for 15-30 seconds and repeat on the opposite side.

Chest and Back Stretches

1. Doorway

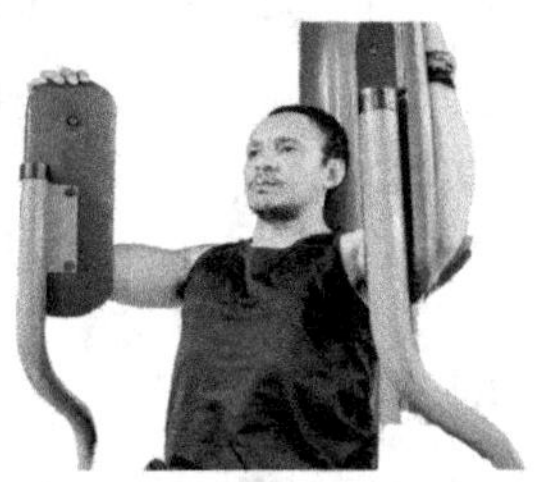

Chest Stretch

Stand facing a doorway and lay your forearms on either side of the door frame. Step forward with one foot to create a slight stretch in the chest. Hold for 15-30 seconds.

2. Upper Back Stretch

Sit on a chair and

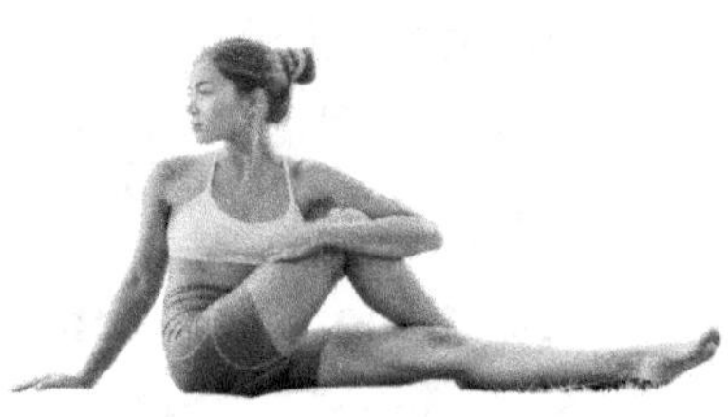

cross one leg over the other. Twist your torso in the opposite direction, placing one hand on the outside thigh for support. Hold the stretch for 15-30 seconds and repeat on the opposite side.

3. Child's Pose

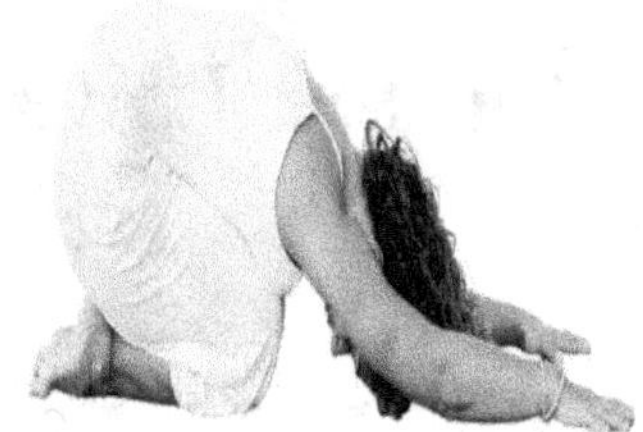

Begin with your hands and knees, then sit back on your heels while lowering your chest toward the floor.

Extend your arms forward and rest your forehead on the ground.

Feel the stretch in your back and hold for 15-30 seconds.

4. Cat-Cow Stretch

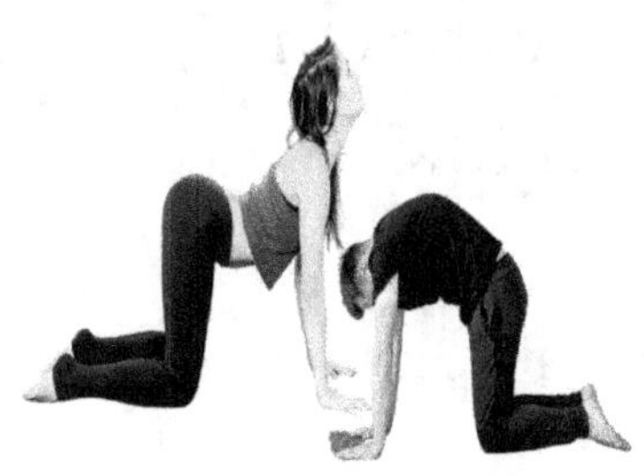

Start on your hands and knees, then gently arch your back upward, dropping your head and tailbone. Hold for a few seconds, then drop your tummy and lift your head and tailbone, making a little bend in the back. Repeat for multiple repetitions.

Stretching Exercises for the Lower Body

Maintaining flexibility in the lower body is vital for seniors to enhance mobility, reduce accidents, and improve the overall quality of life. Stretching exercises targeted towards the lower body can assist improve the range of motion in the hips, legs, and feet, allowing for better freedom of movement.

In this part, we will explore a range of stretching exercises intended exclusively for the lower body. From stretching the hamstrings and quadriceps to the calves and hip flexors, these exercises will enhance flexibility and help elderly maintain optimal lower body function.

Leg Stretches

1. Hamstring Stretch

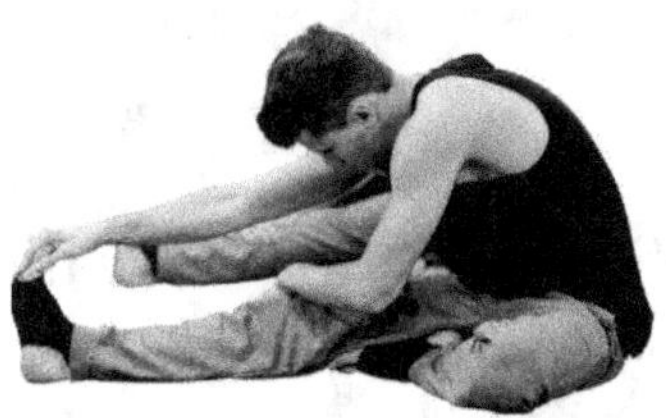

Sit on the floor with one leg extended in front of you and the other leg bent. Lean forward from your hips, reaching towards your extended foot while keeping your back straight. Feel the stretch in the back of your thigh. Hold for 15-30 seconds and repeat with the other leg.

2. Quadriceps Stretch

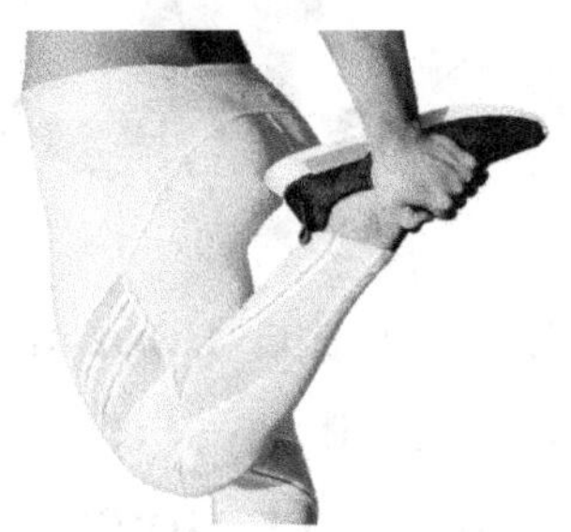

Stand near a wall or chair for support. Bend one leg at the knee and grip your ankle, bringing your heel towards your buttocks. Feel the stretch in the front of your thigh. Hold for 15-30 seconds and swap legs.

3. Inner Thigh Stretch

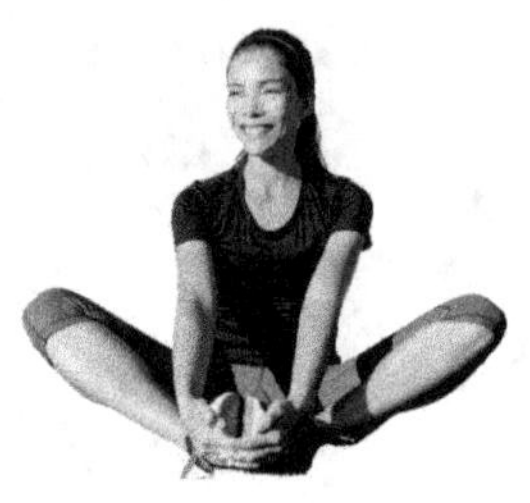

Sit on the floor and bring the soles of your feet together. Hold your ankles and slowly press your knees toward the floor. Feel the stretch in your inner thighs.

Hold for 15-30 seconds.

4. Calf Stretch

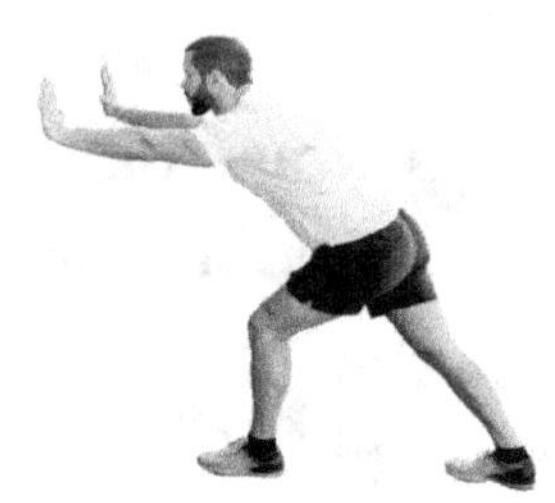

Stand facing a wall and place your hands on it for support. Step one foot back, keeping it straight with the heel on the ground. Lean forward, experiencing the strain in your calf muscle. Hold for 15-30 seconds and swap legs.

Hip Stretches

1. Hip Flexor Stretch
Kneel on one knee with the other foot in front of you. Gently thrust your hips forward, feeling the 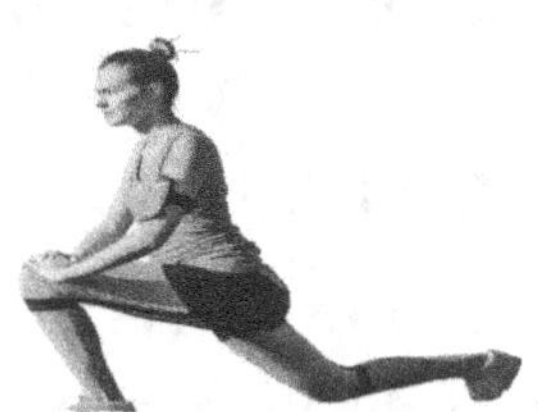 stretch in the front of your hip. Hold for 15-30 seconds and switch sides.

2. Pigeon Pose
Start in a push-up position, then bring one knee 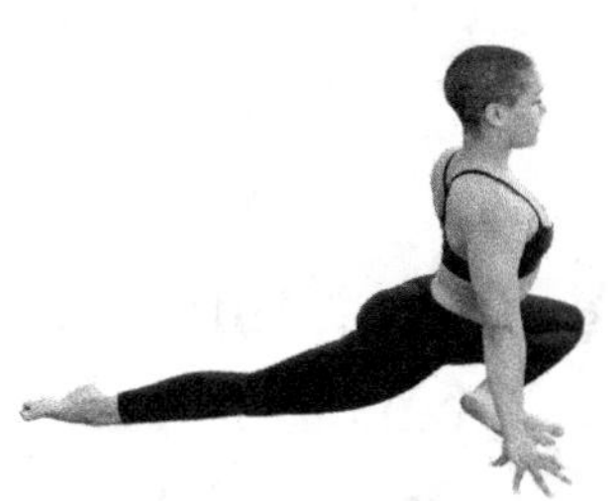 forward and place it on the ground, slanted out to the side. Slide the second leg back, keeping it straight. Lean forward, feeling the stretch in your hip. Hold for 15-30 seconds and switch sides.

3. Seated Hip Stretch

Sit on the edge of a chair with one ankle crossed over the opposing knee. Gently press down on the crossed knee, feeling the stretch in your hip. Hold for 15-30 seconds and swap legs.

Ankle and Foot Stretches

1. Toe Curls

Sit in a chair and place a towel on the floor in front of you. Use your toes to grab and scrunch the towel, then release. Repeat multiple times to stretch and strengthen the muscles in your feet.

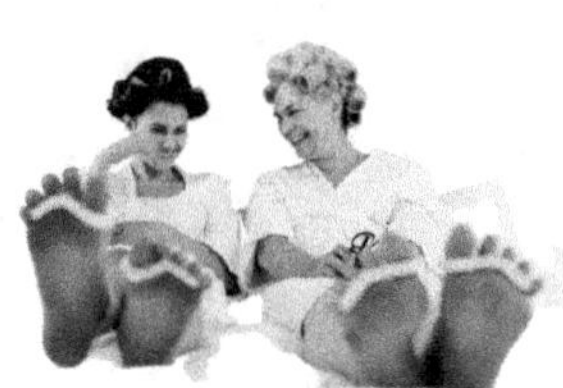

2. Ankle Circles

Sit on the floor with your legs extended. Lift one leg and rotate your ankle in a circular motion. Repeat in the opposite direction. Perform 10-15 circles in each direction, then switch to the other leg.

3. Plantar Fascia Stretch

Stand facing a wall and place your hands on it 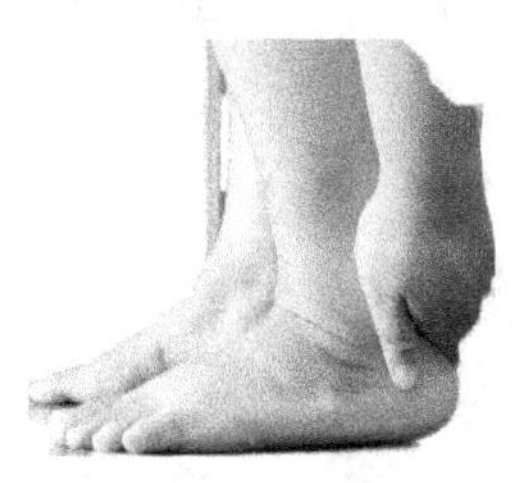 for support. Step one foot back and maintain the heel on the ground. Gently lean forward, feeling the stretch at the bottom of your foot. Hold for 15-30 seconds and switch sides.

Incorporating these leg, hip, ankle, and foot exercises into your normal regimen will help increase flexibility, reduce muscular tension, and support lower body mobility. Remember to practice these stretches slowly and within a comfortable range of motion. If you have any current injuries or medical concerns, contact a healthcare practitioner before performing these workouts.

Chapter 3

Stretching Routines for Specific Conditions

Stretching regimens suited to individual situations can play a key role in controlling and improving overall well-being. Whether you're battling with arthritis, osteoporosis, or chronic pain, targeted stretching exercises can help alleviate symptoms, increase flexibility, and enhance functional capacity.

In this chapter, we will investigate stretching exercises developed for certain conditions. These routines take into account the special demands and limitations of persons with certain health conditions, providing safe and effective exercises to increase strength, flexibility, and mobility. By implementing these stretching practices into your daily regimen, you may empower yourself to take an active role in controlling your condition and maintaining a healthier, more active lifestyle.

Exercises for Arthritis and Joint Pain

1. Range of Motion Exercises: Gently exercise each affected joint through its complete range of motion, such as shoulder circles, wrist bends, and ankle rotations. Perform these exercises every day to maintain flexibility and reduce stiffness.

2. Low-Impact Aerobic Activities: Engage in low-impact workouts like walking, swimming, or cycling to increase joint flexibility, reduce discomfort, and enhance overall cardiovascular health. Start with shorter durations and progressively increase as tolerated.

3. Strength Training: Incorporate modest resistance workouts to strengthen the muscles surrounding the afflicted joints. Use tension bands or modest weights to do workouts like bicep curls, leg presses, and shoulder lifts. Start with lighter weights and progressively progress.

Exercises for Osteoporosis and Bone Health

1. Weight-Bearing Exercises: Engage in weight-bearing activities that exert stress on bones, such as walking, dancing, or stair climbing. These activities assist maintaining bone density and strengthen bones.

2. Balance Exercises: Perform balance exercises including standing on one leg, heel-to-toe walk, or yoga poses like tree pose. These exercises increase balance and stability,

minimizing the incidence of falls and fractures.

3. Strength Training: Include resistance workouts that target major muscle groups to help build bones and prevent additional bone loss. Examples include squats, lunges, and modified push-ups.

Exercises for Balance and Fall Prevention

1. Standing Leg Lifts
Stand behind a chair and lift one leg to the side, front, and back. Hold each position for a few seconds. Gradually increase the duration and repetitions as your balance improves.

2. Toe-to-Heel Walk
Walk in a straight line, placing your heel directly in front of the toes of the opposing foot with each stride. This exercise helps enhance balance and coordination.

3. Tai Chi

Practice tai chi, a graceful and flowing martial art that stresses balance, coordination, and mindfulness. Tai chi can assist enhance balance, flexibility, and total body control.

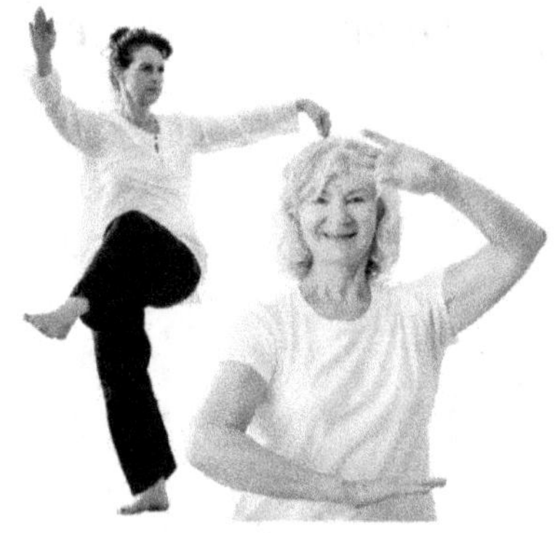

Stretching for Everyday Activities

Stretching is not only good for dedicated exercise or training sessions but also plays a significant part in everyday activities. From reaching for goods on high shelves to bending down to tie your shoes, flexibility, and mobility are vital for doing daily chores with ease and avoiding the risk of injury.

In this part, we will explore the relevance of stretching for everyday tasks and present practical ideas on incorporating stretching into your daily routine. By knowing the benefits and incorporating stretching exercises into your everyday life, you can strengthen your overall physical capabilities and improve your quality of life.

Stretching for Walking and Mobility

1. Quadriceps Stretch

Stand near a wall or chair for support. Bend one leg at the knee and grip your ankle, bringing your heel towards your buttocks. Feel the stretch in the front of your thigh. Hold for 15-30 seconds and swap legs. This stretch focuses on the quadriceps muscles, which are vital for walking and maintaining leg strength.

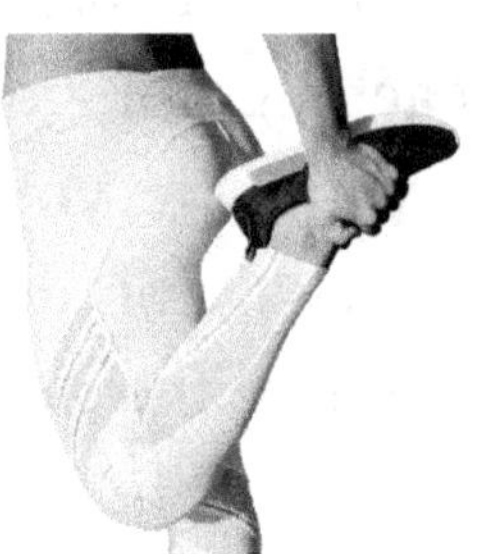

2. Hip Flexor Stretch

Kneel on one knee with the other foot in front of you. Gently thrust your hips forward, feeling the stretch in the front of your hip. Hold for 15-30 seconds and switch

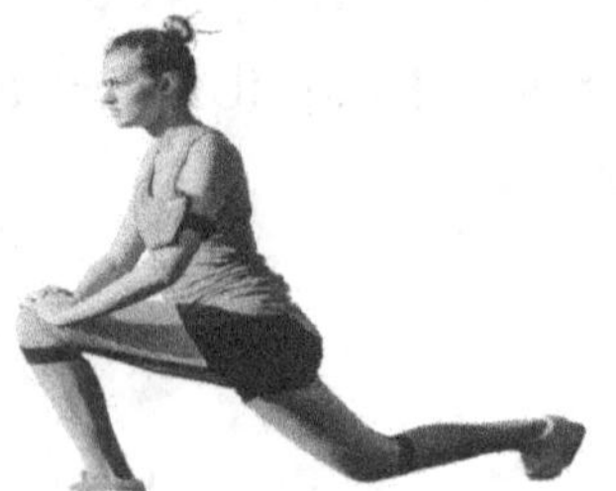

sides. This stretch helps reduce stiffness in the hip flexor muscles, allowing for greater walking and mobility.

3. Ankle Rolls

Sit on a chair and elevate one foot off the ground. Rotate your ankle in clockwise and counterclockwise circles. Perform 10-15 circles in each direction, then switch to the other foot. Ankle rolls can enhance ankle mobility, aiding in walking and keeping balance.

Stretching for Sitting and Desk Work

1. Neck Stretch

Sit tall in your chair and slowly tilt your head to one side, bringing your ear towards your shoulder. Hold for 15-30 seconds and repeat on the opposite side. This stretch helps reduce tension in the neck muscles frequently induced by extended sitting and desk work.

2. Upper Back Stretch

Sit on the edge of your chair and interlace your fingers in front of you. Round your upper back, stretching your arms forward while pressing your shoulder blades apart. Hold for 15-30 seconds. This stretch helps overcome the slumped posture associated with sitting and desk work.

3. Wrist and Finger Stretches

Extend one arm forward with the palm pointing down. Use your other hand to gently draw the fingers back towards your body. Hold for 15-30 seconds and repeat on the opposite hand. This stretch helps ease stiffness and tightness in the wrists and fingers produced by typing and mouse use.

Stretching for Gardening and Household Chores

1. Standing Side Bend

Stand with your feet

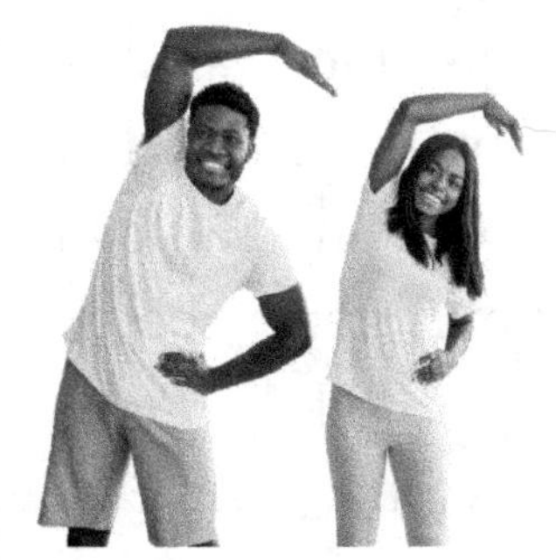

hip-width apart and lay your hands on your hips. Gently bend to one side, feeling the stretch in your torso. Hold for 15-30 seconds and repeat on the opposite side. This stretch helps prepare your body for reaching, lifting, and bending while gardening and home activities.

2. Lunge Stretch

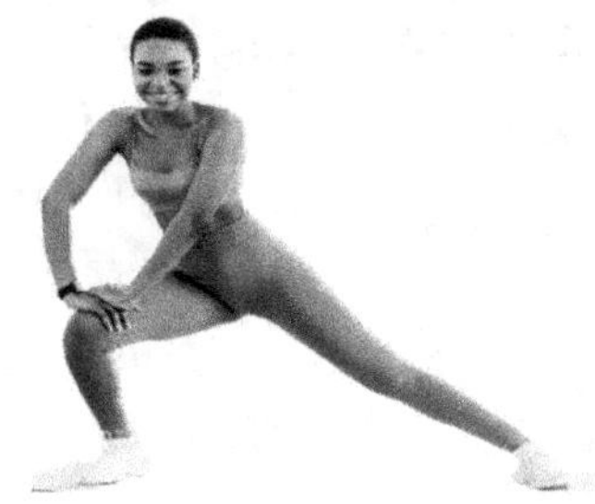

Step one foot forward into a lunge position, with your knee bent and your back leg straight.

Place your hands on your front thigh for support. Lean forward slightly, experiencing the stretch in your hip flexors and thighs. Hold for 15-30 seconds and switch sides. This stretch prepares your body for activities like squatting, kneeling, and reaching while gardening and doing chores.

3. Standing Forward Fold

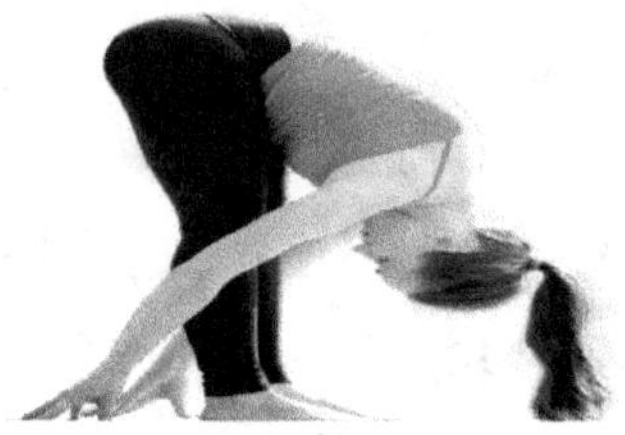

Stand with your feet hip-width apart and slowly bend forward at the hips, allowing your upper body to hang lightly. Feel the stretch in your hamstrings and lower back. Hold for 15-30 seconds. This stretch helps release tension in the lower back and hamstrings, which can become tight during activities like gardening and domestic tasks

Chapter 4

Partner Stretches and Assisted Stretching

Stretching is not limited to solitary efforts but can also be boosted through partner stretches and aided stretching techniques. Partner stretches use the assistance of another person to allow deeper stretches and target specific muscle areas that are difficult to reach on your own.

Assisted stretching, on the other hand, involves the use of props or instruments to assist in obtaining optimal stretching positions.

In this chapter, we will discuss the benefits and practices of partner stretches and assisted stretching, showing how these methods can strengthen flexibility, improve range of motion, and create deeper relaxation. Whether you have a workout partner or seek the help of a trained professional, including partner stretches and assisted stretching into your regimen can take your flexibility journey to new heights.

Partner Stretches for Seniors

1. Seated Back Stretch

Sit on the floor facing your partner with your legs extended in front of you. Reach forward and clasp hands with your partner, gently pulling

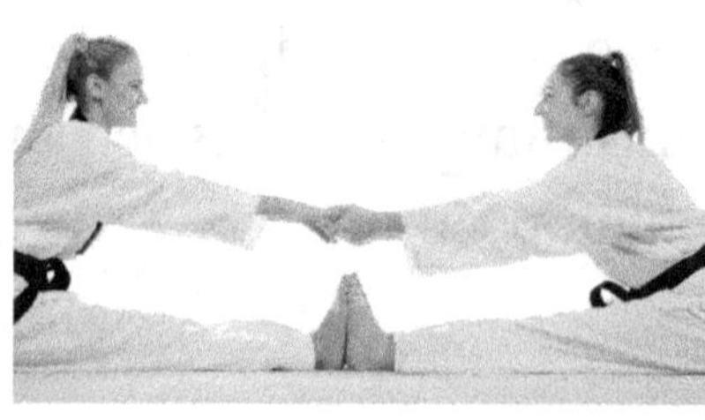

forward to extend your back. Hold the stretch for 15-30 seconds while keeping a relaxed breathing rhythm.

This stretch helps increase flexibility in the back and shoulders.

2. Standing Quadriceps Stretch

Stand facing your partner, holding onto their shoulder or forearm for support. Bend one knee and bring your foot towards your buttocks, with your partner assisting in maintaining balance. Hold the stretch for 15-30 seconds and switch sides. This stretch targets the quadriceps muscles and increases leg flexibility.

3. Seated Hamstring Stretch

Sit on the floor with your legs extended in front of you and your partner seated behind you. Extend one leg forward while your partner softly presses on your shoulders, allowing you to lean forward. Hold the stretch for 15-30 seconds and swap legs. This stretch helps enhance flexibility in the hamstrings.

4. Standing Chest Opener

Stand back-to-back with your partner and interlace your arms at the elbows. Slowly walk away from each other while maintaining your arms interlaced, feeling a stretch in your chest and shoulders. Hold the stretch for 15-30 seconds. This stretch helps enhance chest and shoulder mobility.

Assisted Stretching Techniques

1. Strap-Assisted Hamstring Stretch

Lie on your back and loop a strap or towel around the ball of one foot. Extend your leg upward with the strap, maintaining your knee straight. Your companion can assist in gently pulling the strap to deepen the stretch. Hold for 15-30 seconds and swap legs. This stretch targets the hamstrings.

2. Wall-Assisted Calf Stretch

Stand facing a wall and place your hands on the wall for support. Step one foot back and maintain the heel on the ground. Your spouse can offer light pressure on your calf to increase the stretch. Hold for 15-30 seconds and swap legs. This stretch helps increase calf flexibility.

3. Chair-Assisted Hip Flexor Stretch

Stand facing a sturdy chair and place one foot on the chair seat with the knee bent at a 90-degree angle. Your companion can aid in gently pressing down on your hip, intensifying the stretch at the front of your hip. Hold for 15-30 seconds and swap legs. This stretch targets the hip flexor muscles.

Partner stretches and assisted stretching techniques provide additional assistance, encouragement, and a deeper level of stretching that may not be feasible on your own. Remember to communicate with your spouse and avoid pushing beyond your comfort level. These exercises can boost flexibility, improve range of motion, and promote relaxation, making them ideal compliments to a senior's stretching program.

Stretching and Relaxation

Stretching and relaxing go hand in hand, providing a strong combination that enhances total well-being. Stretching not only enhances flexibility and mobility but also allows for profound relaxation of both the body and mind.

In this part, we will investigate the connection between stretching and relaxation, and how including stretching into your routine can help you achieve a sense of tranquility and quiet.

Stretching for Stress Relief

1. Deep Breathing Stretch

Start by taking a deep breath in, then as you exhale, slowly stretch your arms aloft and reach towards the sky. Feel the stretching of your spine and the opening of your chest. Hold the stretch for a few breaths, allowing tension to dissipate with each exhale. This stretch helps induce relaxation and decreases tension.

2. Seated Forward Fold

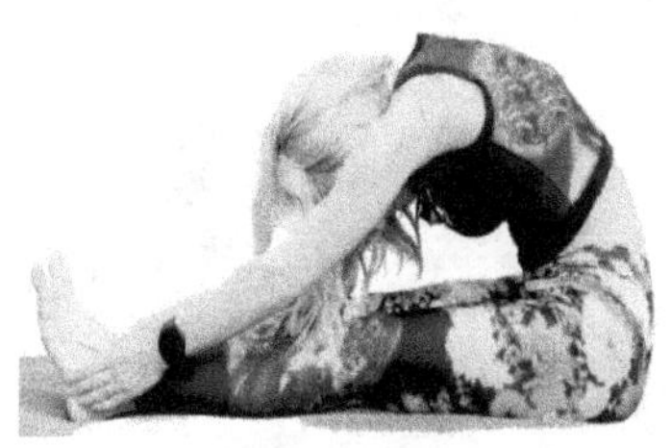

Sit on the floor with your legs extended in front of you. Slowly fold forward from your hips, reaching towards your toes or ankles. Aas you fold, focus on breathing deeply and letting go of tension in your back and hamstrings.

Hold the stretch for several breaths, feeling a sense of release and relaxation.

3. Child's Pose

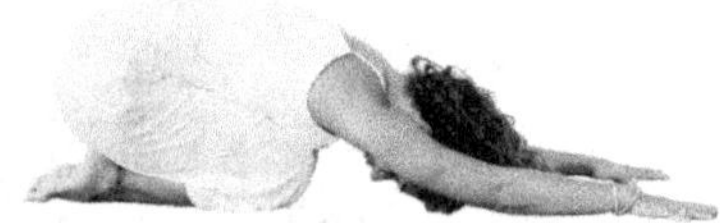

Begin by kneeling on the floor and then softly drop your buttocks towards your heels. Extend your arms forward and rest your forehead on the mat or a cushion. Breathe deeply and allow your body to sink into the pose, releasing tension from your back, shoulders, and neck. Stay in this stance for several breaths, feeling a sense of tranquility.

4. Standing Side Stretch

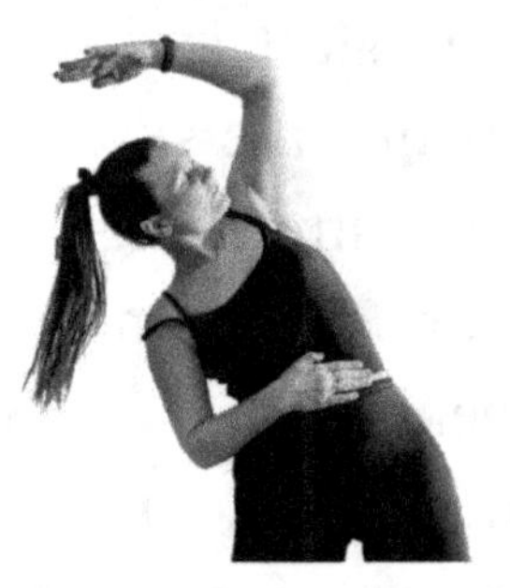

Stand tall with your feet hip-width apart. Extend one arm overhead and slowly lean to the opposite side, experiencing a stretch along your side body. Breathe deeply and hold the stretch for a few breaths. Repeat on the other side. This stretch helps release tension in the neck, shoulders, and torso, promoting relaxation.

Chapter 5

Incorporating Mindfulness into Stretching

Mindfulness means being fully present at the moment and fostering a non-judgmental awareness of your thoughts, sensations, and environment. Here are some methods to include mindfulness in your stretching routine:

1. Focus on Sensations: Pay attention to the bodily sensations you experience with each stretch. Notice the sense of your muscles stretching, the warmth or coolness in your body, and the breath moving in and out. Stay present in the sensations without judgment or distractions.

2. Practice Deep Breathing: Use your breath as an anchor to pull yourself into the present moment. Take calm, deep breaths as you proceed through each stretch. Focus on the inhalation and exhalation, allowing the breath to direct your movements and build a sense of peace.

3. Let Go of Thoughts: During stretching, thoughts and distractions may arise. Instead of getting caught up in them, acknowledge them and gently let them go. Bring your attention back to the present moment, to the feelings in your body and the flow of your breath.

Take the time to calm down, be present, and appreciate the harmonious balance of stretching and mindfulness in your daily routine.

Designing a Personalized Stretching Program

Designing a customized stretching routine is a critical step toward increasing your flexibility, mobility, and overall physical well-being. While standard stretching routines give many benefits, adapting a program to your unique requirements and goals can take your development to new heights.

In this part, we will explore the importance of a customized stretching program and provide information on how to develop one that meets your specific needs. By recognizing your body's strengths, weaknesses, and restrictions, and by using a range of stretching techniques and exercises, you can develop a program that addresses your specific areas of concentration and helps you reach optimal results.

Get ready to go on a voyage of self-discovery and develop a stretching routine that will complement your body's demands and unlock your maximum potential.

Setting Goals and Tracking Progress

When it comes to establishing a personalized stretching program, setting objectives and tracking progress are vital for remaining motivated and attaining success. By establishing precise objectives, you may adapt your program to reach particular targets and monitor your success along the way. Here are some ways to help you set objectives and properly track your stretching journey:

1. Define Your Goals: Start by establishing what you want to achieve with your stretching routine. It could be improving flexibility in select regions, increasing the range of motion, reducing muscle tightness, or promoting

general mobility. Be explicit and practical with your goals.

2. Break Down Goals into Milestones: Breaking your major goals into smaller, realistic milestones can assist retain concentration and drive. Set short-term targets that guide you toward your ultimate purpose. For example, if you aim to touch your toes, establish a milestone to reach a given distance from your knees within a specified timeframe.

3. Track Your Progress: Keep a diary of your stretching sessions, including the exercises performed, duration, intensity, and any remarks. This log will help you monitor your development and find patterns or adjustments needed in your routine. Consider utilizing a notebook, a mobile app, or an online tracker to chronicle your sessions conveniently.

4. Assess and Adjust: Regularly assess your progress to determine if you are coming closer to your goals. Evaluate your flexibility, range

of motion, and overall comfort throughout activities. If needed, make adjustments to your program, such as increasing the time or severity of stretches, introducing new exercises, or adjusting the frequency of your sessions.

Modifying Exercises for Individual Needs

Each person is unique, and their bodies have various capabilities, weaknesses, and conditions. Therefore, it is necessary to customize stretching exercises to fit individual demands. Here are some considerations for adjusting workouts in your personalized stretching program:

1. Physical restrictions: If you have any existing injuries, chronic diseases, or physical restrictions, it is vital to adapt activities properly. Consult with a healthcare practitioner or a trained trainer who can assist with changes that will be safe and beneficial for your circumstances.

2. Flexibility Levels: Modify stretches based on your current flexibility levels. If you are a beginner or have limited flexibility in a particular area, start with softer variations of the exercises and progressively increase as your flexibility improves. Listen to your body and avoid going beyond your comfort zone to prevent injury.

3. Range of Motion: Adjust exercises to accommodate your range of motion. For instance, if you have limited shoulder mobility, you can use a towel or strap to increase your reach during stretches. Props and tools can assist in obtaining proper alignment and support, allowing you to safely explore your full potential.

4. Personal tastes: Take into account your tastes and interests when building your program. If you find particular activities more fun or effective, prioritize incorporating them into your routine. Enjoying your stretching

routine boosts adherence and makes it a more pleasant experience.

Conclusion

Frequently asked questions

Can I Stretch if I Have Certain Health Conditions?

Stretching can be beneficial for many persons with various health concerns, but it is vital to discuss it with your healthcare practitioner before starting any stretching program. Certain health issues may necessitate changes or particular instructions to guarantee safety and effectiveness.

Your healthcare professional can analyze your condition, make recommendations, and guide you on the right stretches or changes that fit your unique needs and restrictions. They can also help evaluate whether any precautions or limits are warranted based on your health condition.

How Often Should I Stretch?

The frequency of stretching depends on various things, including your goals, present flexibility level, and general physical activity. Generally, it is advisable to incorporate stretching into your routine at least two to three times per week.

However, if your goal is to enhance flexibility or treat specific areas of tightness, more regular stretching sessions may be beneficial. Listen to your body and avoid overstretching, as this can lead to injury. It's crucial to establish a balance that works for you and talk with a healthcare practitioner or a competent trainer to decide the proper frequency based on your unique circumstances.

Can I Stretch if I've Had Joint Replacement Surgery?

If you have undergone joint replacement surgery, it is vital to follow your surgeon's post-operative guidelines and suggestions for stretching and physical activity. In many circumstances, stretching can be a crucial element of the recovery process after joint replacement surgery.

However, the particular rules may vary depending on the type of surgery, the joint involved, and your healing status. Your healthcare physician or physical therapist will give you exercises and stretches that are safe and appropriate for your situation. It is vital to stick to their recommendations and report any discomfort or concerns you may have during the stretching procedure.

Scan the code to join our 30 day workout challenge also access Stretching Video training for seniors

***How To Scan**

4. Navigate to your phone Camera or QR Code Scanner app
5. Centre the code in the space given
6. With your mobile data on you'll be directed to the bonus site.

Exercise Plan For Seniors

Quick and Easy Senior Stretching Exercise Plan

1. Neck Stretch:
   - Gently tilt your head to one side, holding for 15 seconds.
   - Repeat on the other side.

2. Shoulder Roll:
   - Roll your shoulders forward in a circular motion for 10 seconds.
   - Reverse and roll them backward for another 10 seconds.

3. Arm Reach:
   - Extend one arm overhead and reach to the opposite side.
   - Hold for 15 seconds, then switch arms.

4. Wrist and Ankle Circles:
   - Rotate your wrists clockwise and counterclockwise for 10 seconds each.
   - Do the same with your ankles.

5. Chest Opener:
   - Sit or stand with good posture.
   - Clasp your hands behind your back, opening your chest and holding for 15 seconds.

6. Seated Leg Stretch:
   - Sit on the edge of a chair and extend one leg
straight.
   - Gently reach for your toes, holding for 15 seconds.
   - Switch legs.

7. Standing Calf Stretch:
   - Stand facing a wall, placing your hands on it.
   - Step one foot back, keeping it straight, and press the
heel into the floor.
   - Hold for 15 seconds, then switch legs.

8. Gentle Torso Twist:
   - Sit or stand with your back straight.
   - Twist your torso to one side, holding for 15 seconds.
   - Repeat on the other side.

Remember to breathe deeply and consistently during
each stretch. If you experience pain, stop and consult
with a healthcare professional before continuing. Enjoy
your stretching routine!